WALK THIN

INTRODUCTION TO WALKING: WHY WALKING IS AN EXCELLENT EXERCISE

Whether searching for a fool-proof strategy for losing weight or a fitness program that is guaranteed to improve your overall health, walking may be the best way to get the results that you're seeking. This exercise is low-impact and capable of burning a considerable amount of fat and calories. There is minimal risk of injury and the opportunity to dramatically reshape and redefine your physique. In fact, this is one of the best exercises for blasting abdominal fat, reducing stress hormones and gaining mood balance. The benefits of taking daily walks, however, extend far beyond these.

Stave Off Age-Related Disease and a Variety of Common Health Issues

Walking for just thirty minutes per day can have a marked impact on your blood pressure. In fact, this is the easiest way to lower blood pressure levels all-naturally. A short walk at a moderate pace can serve as a tremendous form of stress-relief by giving people time to quiet their thoughts, solve problems or reflect on things that they are grateful for. These experiences are both meditative and cathartic and thus, those who take regular walks tend to have fewer blood pressure and heart health issues and far less stress. Surprisingly, moderate walks can also help to alleviate the joint discomfort and swelling caused by arthritis. Thus, getting active is one of the best ways to start feeling better when plagued by stress and physical aches and pains.

Reduce Chronic Anxiety and Depression

One of the top reasons why walking is an excellent exercise is its ability to fight off chronic depression and anxiety. This is especially true for those who opt to take their walks outdoors. Fresh air and sunshine can lend new perspective to even an unwavering pessimist. Moreover, the alternate arm and leg movements that walking entails help to stimulate increased brain activity and improved circulation. Thirty minutes or more of long, rapid strides can boost serotonin levels, flood the body with endorphins and eliminate stress hormones.

Say Goodbye to Excess Cortisol and Watch Your Waistline Shrink

People who struggle with excess belly fat often do so because they are constantly under stress. Cortisol is a stress hormone that serves as the key contributor to the storage of excess fat around the mid-section. Raising the level of endorphins in your body by engaging in routine and moderate exercise is a fast and natural strategy for lowering your cortisol levels. Additionally, by walking, you can boost your metabolism and burn more fat and calories all throughout the day. When it comes to creating a tight, trim abdomen, this is the easiest method.

What many people don't know is that walking is a total body exercise, especially when it is done at a rapid rate. Power walking or advanced walking allows people to build to speeds of 4.5 miles per hour or more. Not only will they be burning approximately 400 calories per hour at this rate, but they will also strengthening their abdominal muscles, tightening their buttocks and toning their arms and thighs. With each step, both the abs and the glutes will be fully engaged. Every comprehensive workout program contains elements of both cardiovascular training and strength training. Power walking is an effective way to get both your strength training and your cardio exercise done in a minimal amount of time.

Overhaul Your Eating Habits

Dieters are often riddled with stress, guilt and frustration. Passing up on fatty foods can be far more challenging when people start these efforts with a heavy sense of defeat. A weight loss program that is centered around moderate exercise, however, can be very empowering. With each step that you take, you can bolster your self-esteem, build your willpower and develop a greater belief in your ability to reach your health and fitness goals. People who use walking for weight loss tend to find it far easier to make common sense-based adjustments to their diets after having experienced workout success, than if relying on dieting alone to drop pounds.

Drop Pounds Regularly

The obvious benefit of walking for weight loss and better health is the fact that you can start melting pounds off with a very minimal amount of effort. This is especially true for walkers who commit to taking 10,000 steps during each session. This is about five miles or one hour and fifteen minutes of walking. With a good pedometer, a sensible pair of walking shoes and a willingness to push towards increased walking speeds and distances, anyone can successfully implement a 10,000 step plan. Not only is this a great way to lose weight, but it is also the surest strategy for keeping it off. Best of all, people will experience higher levels of brain functioning, reduced stress and improved self-confidence along the way.

HOW TO WARM UP, STRETCH AND PREPARE YOUR WALK. INCLUDING IMPORTANT WALKING GEAR

Walking to get from place to place or to gain peace of mind is quite a bit different from walking to burn fat and drop pounds. By committing yourself to taking 10,000 steps each time you workout, you can forever change your life. This common sense and low-risk approach to weight loss is guaranteed to tone up your legs, abdominal muscles and buttocks. It will also shred fat, boost your sense of well-being and flood your system with endorphins. Getting properly dressed and prepared for this process is therefore essential for getting optimal results.

Start With Your Feet

Although walking for weight loss is a relatively low-impact activity, it is still important to pamper and prepare your feet. Depending upon your stride length, 10,000 steps will require you to travel approximately 5 miles. This is a distance that most people take between 60 to 80 minutes to travel and thus, you want to make sure that your feet are ready for this journey. Good walking shoes can be quite a bit different from good running shoes, given the different ways that people move their bodies during these two activities. The ways in which the joints and muscles are used in walking are quite different from the way that they are used when jogging or running. These differences must be reflected in the style of the shoe and in the type and amount of support that is provided.

Runners bend their knees at a greater angle than walkers do. Moreover, their movements are often characterized by small, vertical bounds, rather than a fluid and wholly horizontal stride. Power walking and even walking at a more moderate pace requires a lightweight shoe with a considerable amount of interior cushioning. These should be roomy enough to account for any swelling that might occur, especially for those who are just moving out of a long-term and very sedentary lifestyle.

While runners strike the ground with their forefoot, walkers strike first with the heel and then roll through the ball of the foot to push off the toes. This movement requires good mobility for the mid-portion or ball of the foot. Thus, it is vital to look for options that have flexible soles. You should additionally shop for designs that provide adequate traction and that are made from materials that supply plenty of ventilation.

Choosing a Pedometer

A good pedometer is likely the most important piece of walking gear that people can invest in. This device counts the number of strides that are taken during each walking session. Given that the total walking distance for 10,000 strides will vary according to leg length and stride length, it is better to calculate your walking distance with the use of a trusty pedometer, rather than attempting to tackle a five mile course. Moreover, using a pedometer will help you to determine your maximum walking distance and your maximum walking speed. You can use this data to boost your pace and to push yourself to go farther. More often than not, it will take a new power walker several weeks before he or she is able to complete a full 10,000 strides without stopping for a rest.

There are three types of pedometers that people can choose from. These include hairspring models, coiled spring devices and accelerometers. Among these, hairspring models tend to be the least reliable. In order to get an accurate stride count, these low-cost units will need to be kept in a perfectly upright position and thus, they are less than ideal for long journeys that entail lots of leg movement.

A number of high-end designs will do far more than simply count your steps. These innovative devices can be worn on the wrist and will give accurate readings, no matter how they shift or slide. People can use these to track the total distances that they have walked, see how many calories they have burned, monitor their heart rates and get speed estimates among other things. Walking for weight loss does not require you to invest in one of the most expensive and innovative pedometer designs. You should, however, look for options that will continue to function effectively, even when they move around. Ultimately, you want to invest in a durable option that collects sufficient data for managing your workout and improving your distance and speeds.

Protecting Your Legs

Depending upon the shape of your thighs, it may be necessary to invest in a special type of pants for your workout. Leaving the house in shorts could cause you to suffer from inner thigh chaffing and other friction-related issues. Powering your way through five miles can be excruciating when the insides of your legs have been rubbed raw. When shopping for workout pants, check for materials that will minimize inner-thigh friction while providing adequate airflow. The best options will help to wick moisture away from the skin so that this area stays clean and dry, no matter how hard you push your body.

Warming Up

You might think it's silly to warm up your body up for a walk, but taking a few minutes to loosen up your muscles and elevate your heart rate before getting started can significantly lower your likelihood of sustaining an injury. In fact, it is important to warm up before engaging in any activity that is going to increase your respiration levels. Surprisingly, for these efforts, the best way to get started is by taking a short walk. Rather than pushing yourself to move at maximum speeds, however, just maintain a nice, comfortable stride. After three to four minutes of constant motion, stop and get ready to stretch out. It is never a good idea to start stretching while your muscles are still cold.

Walking, especially advanced walking or power walking, is a whole body exercise. This makes it important to perform stretches that help to loosen and limber up each major muscle group. Start at the top of the head and work your way down so that no muscle group is missed. Stretch the neck, the shoulders, the mid and lower back, the hips, buttocks, thighs and calves. Spend time rolling your ankles in small circles in order to loosen these up as well.

Common Stretching Mistakes

There are a few things that you should never do when stretching your muscles as part of your warm-up routine. Foremost among these is hyper-extending at the knees. This is when your knees bend beyond a ninety degree angle so that they travel beyond the tips of the toes. Any stretch that requires a bent knee should be performed with a bend of ninety degrees or less, pushing beyond this will not provide a deeper stretch.

Pulsing while in a stretching position is also less than ideal. It is far better to lean as deeply into the stretch as possible, while deep breathing. Keeping a constant flow of oxygen to your muscles will help them to limber up and lengthen. After having exhaled, try pushing forward into the stretch a bit more. This slow, but deliberate process will promote muscle elasticity, whereas pulsing motions will not.

Certain stretches require people to bring the head closer to the legs. Although this will intensify the stretch, the best results will come by lowering the torso instead. Craning at the neck does not apply the same amount of tension as lowering the chest will. Thus, when reaching forward to touch your toes while sitting in a pike position, work to bring your chest closer to your knees, rather than your nose. The most important thing to learn about stretching, however, is the proper breathing method. Getting good oxygen delivery is an essential part of this process.

Developing Good Breathing Skills

Any athlete or musician worth his salt can tell you that good respiration begins in the belly. Many people are used to puffing out their chests and raising their shoulders when taking in deep breaths. These movements make them feel as though they are filling their lungs to capacity. In reality, however, this type of breathing is not capable of delivering an optimal flow of oxygen to the body. Rather than concentrating on filling the lungs and letting the shoulders follow through, focus on expanding the diaphragm instead. This is a thick muscle that is horizontally situated between the chest and stomach cavities. To practice diaphragmatic breathing, place the palm of your hand over your stomach. Breathe in while making an effort to move your hand by expanding the diaphragm. There should be minimal expansion in the lungs and no movement in your shoulders.

The Benefits of Diaphragmatic Breathing

Learning how to breathe with the diaphragm is not likely to prove critical during the formative stages of your workout. Once you progress to advanced walking and start moving at a rate that will allow you to traverse 4.5 miles or more in an hour, using diaphragmatic breathing will help you to avoid post-workout soreness and stave off fatigue. It is the best breathing technique to use during an intense workout and it is also a strategy that top athletes have long been using for years as a natural form of performance enhancement. You can always rely on the calming effects of this type of breathing during the warm-up and cool-down phases of your routine.

Concentrated breathing through the expansion and contraction of the diaphragm while stretching helps to change brain wave activity from beta wavelengths, which are characterized by stress, to theta and alpha wavelengths, which are healthier and far more conducive to relaxation. Given the fact that walking is a cathartic and meditative workout, it provides a number of stress-relieving benefits that contribute to the elimination of stubborn belly fat. Using this type of breathing as part of your warm-up will help you to approach these endeavors with a greater level of focus. Moreover, you will be able to rid your body of any excess cortisol, which is a stress hormone and a key contributor to belly fat.

Thus, always take the time to use deep, focused breathing that begins and ends in the diaphragm when preparing for your walking routine. As your skill level increases, try using this breathing style while in motion.

Ready, Set, Go

Once you have warmed up your body and loosened all of your muscles, you can hit the starting line without fear of physical strain and injury. Start out at a comfortable pace and slowly build your speed so that you reach peak walking rate at the mid-point of your workout. If you are walking 10,000 steps, try to reach your highest walking speeds at 5,000 steps and maintain this until you have completed 8,000. You can use the remaining 2,000 steps of your workout to slowly decrease your pace. This is far better for the body than starting and ending at a dead standstill. Once you have reached your final step, prepare to cool-down.

Bringing Your Heart Rate Back Down

Slowly tapering your pace will allow your heart beat to decelerate in a gradual and stress-free fashion. Rapid changes in your rate of movement can trigger stress signals, especially when you are pushing your body its hardest. This is why it is important to work at a peak rate and then slowly reduce your intensity, rather than simply coming to a complete stop.

Revisit your earlier stretching routine to again loosen up your major muscle groups. Rather than starting at the top of the head, however, begin at the feet and slowly work your way up. Use diaphragmatic breathing to keep your stress levels down and deliver an optimal amount of oxygen to your muscles. Loosen up the hips, ankles and wrists through easy, rolling motions.

Ramping Up Your Routine

In addition to increasing your distance and your walking speeds, you can also invest in several tools that will help to increase the intensity of your workout. These strategies work best for people who are able to power through their 10,000 strides at optimal walking speeds without getting out of breath or suffering from any extreme physical fatigue. Once you have developed sufficient endurance for completing this routine with ease, try carrying a small pair of hand weights or strap on a modest pair of ankle weights. If you have opted to complete your workout on the treadmill rather than walking outside, you also have the option of playing around with the incline on your machine. Walking at a higher incline will increase the challenge that is placed on your abdominal muscles, buttocks and thighs and will boost your calorie burning potential considerably.

HOW WALKING 10,000 STEPS MAKES YOU LOSE WEIGHT AND BURN BELLY FAT

It might seem surprising that an act as simple as taking a brisk walk can change your life forever. Although walking is something that people do every day, few individuals recognize the potential of this activity when it comes to shedding pounds and losing belly fat. This low-impact exercise is easy on the joints and guaranteed to provide amazing results. All you need to do is remain consistent in your efforts to take a stroll several times per week.

How Walking 10,000 Steps Makes You Lose Weight

Implementing a strict diet plan and adhering to it without fail is certainly one way to lose weight. Unfortunately, this strategy has proved unsuccessful countless times, given that people often find themselves reaching for the very foods that they must leave behind. Walking, however, is fail-proof way to permanently alter your fitness and nutrition-related habits. It takes minimal effort and does not require any special gym memberships, skills or costly training equipment. All you need is a good pair of walking shoes, a low-cost pedometer and plenty of open road.

While a strict diet is a temporary solution to a long-term problem, a routine exercise program can become a way of life. It may not be possible to forgo your favorite foods day in and day out; however, you do have the ability to walk off the extra pounds that you consume. Thus, rather than feeling guilty each time you indulge in a decadent treat, you can simply lace up your shoes and set out to burn some fat.

10,000 steps might seem like a lot, but it is actually a relatively short distance, especially for those who like the meditative and cathartic benefits of taking a long stroll. 10,000 steps are just under five miles and most people can complete this distance in about one and a half hours of moving at a modest pace. As you increase in strength and physical fitness, it will be possible to up your walking speeds by engaging in advanced walking or power walking. Power walking takes walking for weight loss to the next level. Your routine will become part cardiovascular exercise and part intense strength training. Not only will you burn more fat and calories, but you can also up your walking speeds to approximately 4.5 miles per hour, making it possible to complete your 10,000 steps in just over sixty minutes.

Taking a Common Sense Approach to Weight Loss

This is actually a very common sense approach to weight loss as it gives people goals to strive towards that they are more than capable of meeting. Rather than acting as a constant measurement of your willpower and your ability to say no to food cravings, it is instead an effort to build up self-esteem and to empower you to make the changes that will improve the quality of your life. Most dieters who have experienced the frustration of yo-yo diet plans and fad diets find that it is far easier to take a comfortable stroll, than it is count calories, eliminate entire foods groups and endure countless hours of hunger.

In the process of walking their way towards better health, most people also begin to develop better eating habits. This is largely due to the fact that much of the stress and pressure has been stripped away from the weight loss process. Instead of feeling bad about what they have and have not been able to do, these individuals are able to celebrate their daily accomplishments and have real proof of these due to the changing numbers on their pedometers. It is far more rewarding to watch the numbers on a pedometer cycle upwards, than it is to wait for the numbers on the scale to start moving down.

The Science Behind Walking 10,000 Steps for Weight Loss

Putting the body in motion will always be better for weight loss than efforts to cull calories alone. Using different muscle groups will help to stimulate a robust metabolism, which will in turn boost the body's fat burning abilities. Active individuals tend to burn off more fat and calories while in a state of rest, than those who remain sedentary throughout the day. A brisk walk at your personal, maximum distance and speed can help you to burn between 100 and 200 calories in just thirty minutes. Once you begin power walking your way through the full 10,000 steps, you will be burning in excess of 400 calories per hour. Best of all, your metabolism will continue burning through fats, long after you have cooled your body back down.

Use a Pedometer to Start Increasing Your Distance

It may not be possible to throw yourself headfirst into a five mile walk. There is certainly no shame in that. Most people find that they have to gradually build up to this distance and that it takes several weeks or even months before they can traverse the entire 5 miles with an emphasis on maintaining high speeds. Thus, the best way to get started is by investing in a pedometer. This is a small device that counts the number of steps that you take during each walking session. Simply strap your pedometer on and take your first walk. Take stock of your final walking distance and then try to improve this by 500 steps each time you set out again. If you can only do 2,000 steps on your first try, you can take comfort in the fact that you will be up to 3,000 steps within just a few days. By walking several days per week, you will be able to increase your walking distance by 2,000 to 3,000 steps in almost no time at all.

It is important to note that 10,000 steps is not going to be five miles for all people. This distance is greatly impacted by the length of the individual's stride. Thus, a tall person will actually walk much farther than a person who is of average height or one who is petite. This makes it best to use a pedometer to gauge how far you have walked, rather than attempting to complete a five mile course.

How Walking 10,000 Steps Makes You Lose Belly Fat

Even though it is low-impact and easy to do, walking is actually one of the best whole body exercises. When done properly, walking keeps the abdominal muscles actively engaged. This is especially true when people make a concerted effort to maintain good posture and a brisk walking speed. The unconscious process of drawing the core muscles in will gradually help to slim the waist by building muscle definition and tone in this area. Moreover, with new muscles to support, the body becomes far more likely to draw upon its own fat stores in order to maintain sufficient energy.

It is additionally important to note, however, that the opposite arm and leg movements that walking entails, also helps to firm up and condition the obliques, or the muscles that travel down the side of the body. This is where love handles develop. Thus, if you are tired of carrying around a stubborn spare tire, getting rid of it may be easier than you think. Walking can actually be far more effective for burning belly fat, then endless sit-ups, crunches and other strength-training activities that are performed while lying prone. Best of all, unlike sit-ups, this type of conditioning for the abdominal muscles will not place excess strain on the neck or back.

With stronger core muscles, people can also count on having a much lower likelihood of developing back pain and back injuries. As the central support structure for the body, the spine is heavily reliant upon the core muscles that oppose it. When these are sufficiently strong, people will invariably place less pressure on their lower and mid-backs when moving from one elevation to the next and when lifting and transporting heavy objects.

Tips for Burning Belly Fat Faster

Increasing the length of your strides is certainly one way to start burning larger amounts of belly fat during your routine treks. More importantly, working to build up speed is essential for targeting fat in the abdominal area. Those who walk at a rapid rate are virtually guaranteed to burn off more belly fat than those who walk the same distance, at a more moderate pace.

How It Burns Belly Fat

Power walking or advanced walking causes people to tighten the core muscles and to keep these tightened until they return to a standstill. This type of vigorous exercise combined with a muscle toning element helps to boost the levels of fat burning homes in the body. Thus, not only are you challenging your body to burn off more fat, but you are also altering your chemical composition so that your body becomes and remains perfectly primed for the fat burning process. This means that you are also boosting up the number of calories that your body burns during the post-workout and recovery period, a process that is commonly known as afterburn.

Giving Cortisol the Boot

It certainly doesn't hurt that this type of exercise is also an amazing mood enhancer. Walking for an hour straight gives people the opportunity to quiet down their minds and sort out their pressing problems or escape them. People who constantly feel anxious or tense are prone to storing more belly fat than those who are not. This is because they have higher levels of cortisol, which lends to increased belly fat stores. By engaging in physical activities that diminish anxiety and stress, you can give excess cortisol the boot. Maintaining mood balance and engaging in stress relieving activities is not only important for burning belly fat off, it is also vital for keeping it off for good.

Everything You Need To Know About Power Walking

Once you are ready to start walking long distances at a rapid speed, you need to make sure that you have the right shoes, workout pants and a good pedometer.

The best shoes will give you adequate arch support while allowing for an adequate range of motion in the mid-portion of the foot. Look for pants that reduce friction at the inner thigh, in order to prevent chaffing. It is also a good idea to check for workout gear that has natural wicking capabilities. Once you break a sweat, these articles will draw moisture away from your skin, helping you to stay comfortable longer.

A power walk is not unlike an ordinary walk in that you won't be moving your body vertically. While the next, natural step in the progression of walking speeds would seem like a slow jog, jogging requires you to move your body quite differently. Advanced walking is a pure, horizontal motion with a loose swing of the hips to accommodate the longer gate. This is why joggers experience nearly twice as much pressure on their joints and bones as fast-walkers do. They bound upwards slightly with each step, thereby creating a fusion of both horizontal and vertical motion.

The best way to boost your speeds when using advanced walking to burn more belly fat is by pumping your arms harder. This will make your legs move faster. With each step, make sure that your abdominal muscles and buttocks are fully engaged. This brings the level of intensity that is necessary for increasing your fat burning hormones.

Taking 10,000 Steps for Weight Maintenance

Opting to walk 10,000 steps in a single exercise session might prove challenging on your first several tries. This, however, is one exercise program that few people quit. Efforts to put the body in motion through a low-impact and whole-body activity can have a tremendous impact on how you feel. These jaunts can lift your spirits, alleviate your stress and give you new hope concerning your weight loss goals. People who use this strategy for reducing their body weights and for shedding unwanted belly fat discover that the process of building towards their targeted distances and walking speeds is empowering. As a common sense-based weight loss program, it gives people the chance to set measurable goals that they are capable of achieving. With each new accomplishment, you will feel better able to tackle the other fitness and nutrition-related challenges that lie in your way. Best of all, within just several short weeks you will have created a lifelong habit that will not only produce the results that you have long been waiting for, but that will help you to maintain them as well.

MAKING THE MOST OF YOUR HARD WORK BY CUTTING CALORIES AND ADDING POWERFUL NUTRIENTS. FOOD TIPS

Adopting a workout plan that is the perfect fusion of cardiovascular exercise and strength training is guaranteed to provide visible results. People who use power walking as part of their weight loss programs often drop pounds consistently throughout the first several weeks. In order to avoid troublesome plateaus and get maximum benefits from this type of conditioning, however, it will be necessary to implement the right diet plan. Rather than placing your focus entirely on cutting calories, you should instead work to fuel your body with a comprehensive array of powerful nutrients. The following food tips will show you how.

Foods for Building Lean Muscle Mass

Whether walking at a comfortable pace or using long, rapid strides to power walk your way through your workout, you will be pushing your body to build lean muscle. This new muscle is going to require extra fuel, which is why the metabolism begins to burn off more fat and calories when people incorporate strength training elements into their workout routines. High protein foods will always be the best options for those who are increasing their lean muscle mass, given that protein is the primary building block of muscle. While fats and carbohydrates serve as essential energy sources, protein plays an important role in metabolic functioning and in the development and maintenance of muscle. By eating the right high-protein foods after a grueling workout, you will be giving the body what it needs to replenish and repair the various muscle groups that have been targeted.

Although there are tons of supplements that people can rely on for supplying the body with ample protein, it is always far better to get essential nutrients directly from natural food sources. These will come in forms that the body is able to recognize, effectively break down and absorb. Even some of the highest quality supplements are not able to be fully absorbed by the body and thus, most of these expensive products are often passed back out of the system through the urine and the stool.

Choosing Healthy Protein Sources

There are many ways to start adding larger servings of protein to your diet, even for those who are not fond of meat, fish and other animal-derived protein sources. True nuts, such as almonds, pecans and walnuts are optimal sources of protein as are nut butters, such as almond butter. It is important to note, however, that peanuts are not a true nut and thus, these will deliver far more starch than is ideal for the average weight loss plan.

Legumes are also another important addition to your diet. Black beans, red beans, kidney beans, pinto beans, lentils and chick peas can be used to make soups and other flavorful dishes. These are low in fat and high in protein, making them the perfect way to power up after a grueling workout. Not only are they highly versatile, legumes are also very affordable. In addition to being very protein-dense, they are also rich in magnesium, folate, potassium, iron and soluble fiber. They work to promote heart health and digestive regularity and they can also increase collagen production, which is an essential component of cartilage. Thus, by adding legumes to your diet, you can stave off issues relating to your heart health; avoid constipation while loading your diet with protein and stave off physical injury. Best of all, a meal with legumes will keep you feeling fuller longer, thereby reducing the risk of overeating.

When it comes to meat, lean cuts of white meat are best. Chicken and turkey breast can serve as the basis for nutrient-dense soups, salads and even whole wheat pasta dishes. Several servings of fish per week would be ideal; however, consumers must make careful consideration of their fish suppliers. Wild caught fish is always preferable to farm raised and it is vital to know the regional data on mercury exposure for locally caught seafood.

Identifying Good Carbohydrates

Carbohydrates have been given a bad name over the past few years, given that some of the most popular foods and food products can be responsible for major weight gain. These, however, are essential for maintaining high energy levels and thus, no eating plan is ever complete without them. There is a major difference between natural sources of carbohydrates that nourish and energize the body and those that are heavily refined. Fresh fruits and vegetables are great sources of fuel, given that these are generally low in calories, rich in vitamins and other nutrients and they are very water and fiber dense.

When it comes to grains, you should always look for products that are offered or served closest to their natural state. White flour products have been stripped of most or all of their nutritional benefits and thus, these are often empty calories. Minimizing your intake of empty calorie foods is important, even when you are diligent in maintaining your routine exercise plan. These carbs quickly convert to sugars in the body and can take an extraordinary toll on numerous organ systems. They can also significantly increase the risk of developing diabetes and other weight and nutrition-related health issues.

Steel cut oatmeal is definitely a worthwhile addition to your regular diet. This helps to regulate blood sugar levels and remove toxins from the body. People who are considered to be at high risk for developing diabetes can use this food to move out of the danger zone. Adding cinnamon for taste and sweetening your hot cereal with fresh apple slices, blueberries, blackberries or any other fresh and unprocessed fruit will supply further health benefits. Raw, shelled pecans can even be incorporated into this mix to add a new layer of texture and provide the body with a rich dose of protein. A heart-healthy and complete breakfast like this one is guaranteed to give you the energy that you need for a positive mind-set and a productive day.

Achieving Dietary Balance

The missing ingredient from most weight loss plans is balance. People often develop weight issues by maintaining eating habits that are imbalanced. They eat too many refined carbs, too much sugar and too many of the wrong types of fat. Unfortunately, they attempt to correct this problem by swinging in the opposite direction. Rather than looking for diets that represent a well-balanced blend of all of the essential food groups, dieters routinely cut out major food groups and nutrients thinking that this well help them drop pounds fast.

Deprivation diets can and do produce weight loss, however, these results are rarely guaranteed to last. Once an individual returns to former eating habits, the lost weight is certain to return. Using a deprivation diet for too long can also cause the metabolism to go through a dramatic slow-down. Thus, while your ultimate goal is to cut calories, it is always important to make sure that you are giving your body what it needs. Trying to consume approximately 2,000 calories per day will help you to reach a healthy weight within a reasonable period of time. Moreover, maintaining your new eating patterns will help you to keep the weight off.

Filling Up On Fiber

One of the best strategies for reducing calories is to turn to fresh produce when you feel like snacking. A small handful full of sugar snow peas can provide nearly three times the recommended daily amount of vitamin C. Munching on a crisp apple will clean the teeth, protect the enamel and deliver a potent rush of natural energy. This is far better than relying on processed sandwich breads, snack cakes, chips and cookies, which usually contain a wealth of fat, sugar, sodium and calories while providing the body with minimal benefits.

In addition to being fiber-dense, most fresh fruits and vegetables are also filled with water. This will replenish lost stores after a grueling workout session and will minimize the amount of fresh water that you must drink in order to stay properly hydrated. Ample fruits and vegetables in the diet fosters good digestion and will help to prevent piles, which people often experience after making major changes to their formerly sedentary lifestyles.

Getting Good Fats

Efforts to moderate your intake of fats are important, especially in terms of the amount of high-fat dairy products that you are consuming. While butter, cheese and creams can continue to be a part of your regular diet, you should take care to limit these. The best fats come from nuts, olives and fish. Coconut oil is the ideal cooking oil given its natural anti-fungal and antibacterial properties. It is also a highly stable oil and this means that it can be heated to considerably high heats without undergoing any major chemical changes.

While olive oil has long been lauded as the perfect oil for a healthy diet, it is important to avoid heating or cooking with this oil. Unlike coconut oil, it is highly unstable and its chemical composition will begin to change once it is exposed to high heats. This oil should be used for making salad dressings or for incorporating into other cool or lukewarm dishes, but it should not be used for frying or pan searing.

Making an effort to consume at least one full tablespoon of coconut oil a day can be surprisingly good for your diet. This oil delivers vital nutrients to the brain and is also capable of restoring internal pH levels. For those who have consumed high sugar diets for some time and for people who routinely drink alcoholic beverages, coconut oil can be used to lower high acidity levels and promote weight loss around the midsection. You can use this oil in place of butter by stirring it into your morning oatmeal. It can also be added to hot beverages, soups and other dishes.

Rehydrating the Right Way

Just as giving your body the right types of fats is important for weight loss, choosing the right beverages is vital as well. Once you start kicking your activity levels into high gear, you may be tempted to turn to sports drinks to ensure optimal hydration. Even low-calorie sports drinks, however, can have a detrimental impact on your efforts to attain your health and fitness goals. These products are rife with excess amounts of sodium and sweeteners. With added food coloring and other unhealthy additions, these can actually do more harm than good.

Nothing is better for rehydrating than fresh, pure water. You can add a slice of lemon to this in order to prevent water retention. Adding a few sprinkles of cayenne pepper to a tall glass of warm or cold water will also rev up your metabolism and regulate your blood pressure.

Beyond cold water, it is important to limit your intake of heavily sweetened and highly caffeinated beverages. Diet soda has been shown to be just as bad for the body as full-sugar sodas. In order to get optimal results from your workout, look for pure fruit juices. You can consume several ounces of these per day, along with a full glass of low-fat milk. Coffee or green tea should be fine for a morning beverage, but it is important to limit your use of heavy creamers, flavored syrups, sugar and whipped cream toppings. Swapping out your daily cup of coffee for a small, unsweetened cup of green tea can sometimes produce as much as five pounds of weight loss in a week. Thus, when you find yourself stuck in a rut and unable to drop more pounds, this is definitely a worthwhile change to make.

Treat Yourself to Maintain Motivation and Eliminate Unhealthy Food Cravings

Optimizing your hard work by cutting calories and adding powerful nutrients can certainly have its high points. Some of the most beneficial foods are actually quite delicious. For instance, dark chocolate should become a regular part of your weight loss program. Not only is this a guilt-free way to indulge in a decadent treat, but it can also boost your serotonin levels and reduce your food cravings. Studies have shown that people who eat dark chocolate tend to eat far less than those who deny themselves of sweet, sumptuous fare entirely. Thus, when you feel your weight loss and workout plan starting to fall off track, boost your mood and curb your appetite with a rich square of dark chocolate.

ADVANCED WALKING: BURN MORE CALORIES IN LESS TIME BY POWER WALKING

If you've been walking to drop pounds, you probably think that the next progression in your workout is a move to jogging or running. In reality, however, these high-impact exercises can take a toll on the body that far outweighs the benefits they supply. Thus, the best way to kick your workout plan up a notch is by power walking. Countless fitness experts are extolling the benefits of this low-stress activity. Not only can it help you start burning off more fat and calories in a shorter period of time, but it can also improve brain functioning, alleviate anxiety and improve cognitive thought processes among other things. There is minimal need to worry about getting side-lined by a stress injury and in almost no time you can start looking better, feeling better and functioning better overall.

Getting Geared Up

Avid power walkers make sure to have the right shoes. After all, they will be pushing their bodies a lot harder than if walking at a comfortable stroll. This is basically an activity that lies somewhere between walking and jogging, however, it is important to note that it is often performed at the same speeds. While joggers are hitting the pavement with twice as much force as the average power walker, both of these groups can move equally fast. Thus, the primary difference between advanced walking and jogging is not how fast the body is moving, but rather how it is moving.

Getting a good stride requires loose, flexible footwear that allows for sufficient motion in the mid-range of the foot while providing an optimal amount of arch support. Hard, flat and inflexible soles can cause people to place too much strain on the heels or the shins, given the long and even strides that advanced walking requires. Shoes that are too tight can cause your joints to hurt and make your toes tingle after just a few minutes.

It is additionally important to shop around for footwear options that have great ventilation and interior materials that have natural wicking properties. These will help to keep your feet comfortable even when your body temperature soars and you begin to perspire. The best shoe stores encourage their patrons to spend an ample amount of time moving around in their products. They want to ensure that customers are getting all of the support and mobility that is essential for their chosen activities. Walking enthusiasts should note that the best shoes for a demanding run or a long jog may not be the ideal option for power walking.

Comfortable and motion-appropriate pants are vital as well given that these will help to minimize inner leg friction and the ensuing discomfort. Most workout pants for running or jogging will work well to this end. As you start pumping your arms and legs to build up speed, you don't want to experience the uncomfortable sensation of chaffing.

Warming Up

It generally takes about five minutes to get your heart pumping and your muscles warmed up. Rather than starting a workout session at your fastest speed possible, take some time to gradually build to a decent pace. After five minutes of constant movement, stop and stretch your hamstrings, calves and shoulders. You should also stretch the waist by bending at the upper torso to each side, while keeping the hips stationary. This is a full-body workout which means that you should limber up from your head down to your toes, before getting started with most challenging part of your routine.

Get the Benefits of Strength Training and Cardio Exercise in One Easy Workout

This type of walking requires people to use all of their muscles. This is total body conditioning that burns fat and calories and helps to firm up and tone major muscle groups. When power walking, you should always make sure that your core muscles are engaged. You can do this by imagining that there is a small string attached to your navel and that someone who is slightly taller than you is standing behind you and pulling this string, thereby drawing your navel up and back. When you draw your navel up and in, your abs will be actively engaged. This is how they should stay throughout the duration of your walk.

Although it won't be easy to keep your abdominal muscles fully engaged the first few times that you take a power walk, this is something that is guaranteed to grow easier. With each step, you will be conditioning these muscles and toning them. Your opposite arm and leg movements will help to engage the oblique muscles as well. Before long, you will have a flat, smooth abdomen with an impressive amount of muscle definition.

You should also tighten up your buttocks. It is these efforts that will help you to maximize your body's true fat burning potential. Engagement of the muscles in the abs and buttocks is what transitions this cardiovascular exercise into a challenging strength training routine. Even when moving along a flat and easy plane, you will be developing lots of long, lean muscle. Your body is going to require more calories each day to support this new muscle and thus, your metabolism is going to be moving much faster.

Establish Your Target Speed

The ideal target speed for a good power walk is generally about 4.5 miles per hour. This is similar to a decent jogging speed. Rather than pushing yourself into a slow run, however, you will need to focus on talking long, even strides and on matching your arm movements with your leg movements. There should be a comfortable but moderate sway to your hips in order to allow for greater stride distance and speeds. Rather than gaining air space with each stride and making both vertical and horizontal movements, as with running or jogging, you should be moving horizontally only. If you find yourself bounding off the ground at any point or time, slow down and adjust your stride. Good form is far preferable to high speeds when using advanced walking for weight loss.

As with any moderate-impact activity, it is important to pay attention to your body and how it feels when boosting your walking speeds. While walking at a slow and comfortable pace can burn a significant amount of fat and calories, it will rarely place any major demands on the cardiovascular and respiratory systems. Few people find themselves out of breath when traversing a smooth, level surface and it is not common to break a major sweat or develop an elevated heart rate when walking comfortably. With advanced walking, however, it is not uncommon for people to start feeling winded and fatigued shortly after they start pushing themselves at a much higher pace for the first time. During your first few sessions of power walking, you should pay attention to how your shoes feel, the different areas of your body that are struggling under increased demand and how good it feels to traverse your chosen surface. When moving faster, it could be necessary to take your workout to a track that has a surface with shock absorbing qualities. This is especially true if longer, faster strides cause any discomfort in the hips. Your knees and ankles, however, should not feel any considerable strain if you are moving through your strides correctly.

Building Up To Your Target Speed

Calculating your speed doesn't require any special tools or devices. Simply know how far you are walking and how long it takes you to get there. Divide your waking distance by the number of hours that it takes you to walk this far and this will give you the number of miles per hour that you are traveling. Keeping these calculations simple is a good incentive to push yourself to walk for one full hour, even when starting out. With a good warm-up, this low to moderate-impact exercise is unlikely to cause injury or any extreme measure of post-workout soreness.

As with running or jogging, the fastest and most efficient way to improve your power walking speed is by pumping your arms harder and faster. Your legs will invariably follow suit. It may be difficult to focus on powering through your strides, especially as the buttocks begin to feel the burn of this challenging workout. This is why using the arms to gain speeds is often the best strategy. Given that you can burn more calories in less time with power walking, it is not necessary to push yourself to train for a full hour. People who can, however, will get more mental, physical and emotional benefits from their workouts. These individuals are guaranteed to experience a greater release of endorphins and an optimal amount of stress relief. It is also important to note that the reduced challenge of this activity makes it easier for people to work a lot longer than if jogging or running, even if these individuals are still new to routine exercise. There is always the option to slow down, catch your breath and then push yourself harder once you have the wind and the energy to do so.

Give yourself time to build up to the 4.5 miles per hour pace. This requires you to walk a full mile in approximate 13 minutes, which isn't always an easy feat. Pushing your body to go longer while using the proper form will provide better returns than trying to go fast and burning out after just 20 minutes. At 4.5 miles per hour you can burn off as much as 201 calories in just half an hour. Keeping your body in motion will require the same amount of energy that would be used if your were jogging, thus the number of calories that you burn while protecting your body from energy can be comparable if not better. As your strength and endurance builds, you can move beyond merely pushing yourself to improve your walking speeds. You can start toting a small pair of hand-held weights with you or you can strap on a pair of ankle weights. Walking on a treadmill will additionally give you the option of altering the incline of your walking surface in order to increase or decrease the level of challenge. Thus, there are certainly benefits to performing this exercise indoors during inclement weather.

Pacing Yourself and Cooling Down

If you are able to spend an entire hour walking, you should not be constantly pushing yourself to move at the fastest possible space. The risks of physical injury are best minimized by a power walking plan that includes a gradual increase in speed, a period of peak speeds and then a gradual cool down. Just as you shouldn't start out with your biggest and quickest strides, you shouldn't finish with these either, nor should you come to a dead standstill once your hour is up. Always make sure to spend ten minutes or so bringing your body back down to a slow, steady pace. By the time you stop walking, your heart should be beating slowly and your breathing should have returned to normal. At this time, your muscles will be warm and ready for your post-workout stretching. You should focus on the same muscle groups that were stretched during your warm-up while adding in the buttocks and the abdomen to create a whole body stretching routine. This will help to break up any lactic acid stores and minimize post-workout soreness.

Know Your Motivation

Whether slow and steady or moving at optimal speeds, walking can provide incredible benefits for the brain. In fact, few activities are better than power walking for getting a stimulating rush of endorphins, de-stressing and clearing the mind of clutter. This activity allows for introspection and greater levels of mental peace and calm. More importantly, studies have shown that walking helps to slow mental decline, improves sleep and lowers the risk of Alzheimer's considerably. Walking is also the ideal opportunity to operate with meditative intent, which basically means clearing the brain of external stressors and focusing on breathing and other basic and automatic functions. Many of these are benefits that you can take advantage of right now. Thus, if imagining your ideal body weight is not sufficient for keeping you on track, think about having a better memory, less anxiety or depression and improved cognitive functioning overall.

DEVELOPING THE RIGHT MIND-SET FOR LONG TERM SUCCESS

One of the best things about walking for weight loss is the fact that much of what you need for success will be gradually gained along the way. Taking long walks at a calculated pace is not just good for building muscle, stimulating a robust metabolism and dropping unwanted pounds. These efforts will also help to boost your serotonin levels, flood your body with mood-enhancing endorphins and alleviate a tremendous amount of stress and anxiety. Thus, making a commitment to taking the first steps is the start of gaining the motivation and improved willpower you need for staying on track.

Know What You Want

Defining your goals is critical for weight loss success. This helps people to create realistic expectations for themselves. Setting milestones that are impossible to achieve often causes people to feel frustrated, unmotivated and less than confident. Rather than trying to drop ten pounds over the next two weeks, decide how you want to improve your health overall, reshape your body and tackle your trouble zones. Goals do not always have a specific end, given that they are long-term efforts that will keep you working towards a more superior state of being. Thus, goals can be as simple as lowering or regulating your blood pressure, obtaining and maintaining a healthier body weight, increasing your muscle mass and living an active lifestyle. These are efforts that require gradual but lasting alterations in your life habits, rather than short or sporadic efforts to produce major and immediate changes.

Create Objectives

Objectives are different from goals in that these are small, significant milestones that you can reach which will bring you closer to attaining your goals. Moreover, objectives are quantifiable. For instance, if you want to live a more active lifestyle, then you should establish the objective of walking 10,000 steps per day or roughly the equivalent of five miles, at least three to four times per week. This will not only make you more active, but it will also assist in lowering your blood pressure, balancing your moods and reducing your weight. Dropping 10 pounds can be an objective that will bring you closer to your goal of gaining and maintaining a healthier body weight, however, you should always be careful to give yourself plenty of time to do this. As you increase in physical strength and endurance, you can revisit your objectives to increase the intensity of your workouts. Improving your distance and walking speeds or adding a small pair of hand weights will help you to start moving towards your goals a lot faster.

Get Properly Equipped For Your Workouts

Having what you need for success in your walking for weight loss plan is vital as well. You should have a comfortable pair of walking shoes that provide adequate arch support, a pedometer that functions well in multiple positions and an exercise journal for tracking and recording your process. While you might be eager to start out walking 10,000 steps per day in order to maximize the benefits of these efforts, it will likely take time to build up to this distance. As with all other parts of this process, you should be willing to create feasible objectives that bring your closer to your goal of 10,000 steps. You can use your journal to note how long you were able to walk each day, the pace that you maintained and how you feel about these accomplishments.

Take Note of the Small Improvements

You can also use your journal to record changes that occur in your body that are both positive and unexpected. These are benefits that people may not have been striving for, but which help to boost their life qualities nonetheless. People who walk for weight loss sleep better, respond to stressful situations better, experience digestive regularity and gain marked increases in their muscle tone among many other things. With improved circulation, many individuals also look and feel younger after just several weeks of working out. Appreciating these changes will help you to stay motivated and will keep you committed to the walking schedule that you have created for yourself.

Health Benefits That Might Go Unnoticed

When you have a comprehensive understanding of how walking is capable of altering your body and boosting your overall health, you are much more likely to stick to your plan. Walking, especially advanced walking or power walking, is the perfect, low-impact form of strength training and cardiovascular exercise combined. Walking can help you lose weight, stave off heart disease, moderate stress levels, reduce the stress hormone cortisol, diminish belly fat and keep age-related diseases like osteoarthritis and osteoporosis at bay. Thus, the best way to prepare yourself for long-term success is to minimize your use of the scale and stay focused on your long-term goals. Rather than constantly counting calories and lost pounds, try to remember how these efforts are totally restructuring your life and your life habits overall. With this mind-set, you can stay positive and proactive in your efforts to both bolster and improve your health and fitness levels.

◇◇◇

www.ingramcontent.com/pod-product-compliance
Lightning Source LLC
Chambersburg PA
CBHW061941280526
45787CB00004B/1680